Ashley Fitzgerald

I0416995

WEIGHT LOSS:

GET RID OF FATTENING HABITS AND DONT´DIET ANYMORE

Simple and Easy Ways to Reverse Bad Habits and Lose that Extra Weight

© 2015 by Michael Winicott.
© 2015 by UNITEXTO

Published by UNITEXTO

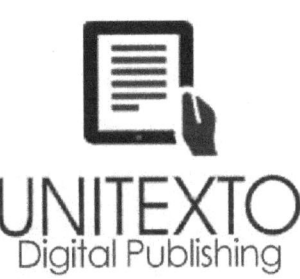

UNITEXTO
Digital Publishing

Table of Contents

Chapter 6: Supplements: Yes or No? (Yes! The right ones)
Green Tea: Energy and Health!
Lemon Water: Oh Yes!
Other Herbs

Chapter 7: Maintain with a Healthy Body and Mind
Replace Bad Habits with Good Habits

Conclusion

Introduction

Behind every bad habit, there's a good habit just waiting to take over and improve your life! Small adjustments can have huge effects on your health, well-being, happiness and overall attitude. It only takes a little motivation, and real desire to change.

Wanting to change is at the core of all successful improvements. You have to realize that things can be better and different, and that the power is in your hands. When you really want to turn things around, that's when the magic happens.

This book will help you get there. It is designed to motivate you, support you, inform you and help you stay patient so that you can finally make your weight loss dreams come true!

Weight loss is not just diet. Nor is it simply about burning off calories. It is about the right integrative lifestyle that comprises both of these factors and more. It's comprehensive, yet simple.

For example, instead of driving to the store, you can try taking a backpack and walking. Once you're there, buy lettuce instead of chips, berries instead of chocolate, fish instead of hamburgers, and so on. You won't feel hungry, but you also won't pig out. The key is to find balance and a way that works for you.

There's no one right way, but we're here to help you change your bad habits around, and make them over into great ones so that you feel inspired and radiant in your life! You will weigh less, have more energy, feel more positive, have a sense of accomplishment, and know that YOUR life is in YOUR hands!

Chapter 1: De-stress and Weigh Less

Do you feel stressed out that you weigh a bit more than you think you should? Relax and ease your mind. Why? Stress is linked to weight gain. Stress produces the hormone cortisol. Cortisol causes the body to store fat, thus leading to weight gain and difficulty in losing weight.

The best thing you can do for yourself is to decide to be healthy because it's good for you. Whatever the circumstances of your life, you can maintain a positive outlook. Of course, it is harder to be positive and feel optimistic when things aren't quite the way you want them to be, you have stress on the job, tension at home, tons of things you need to get done and problems to solve. That's normal.

Fear not. There are some techniques you can employ to reduce your stress so you can get things accomplished without letting it get to you so much that you worry yourself fat. Breathe yourself thin.

Just Breathe

Well, breathing in itself will not make you thin all on its own. But deep, steady breaths are excellent for relaxing the mind and body and supplying energy to all of the cells of the body. This means you will be able to think more clearly. If you are thinking clearly, you will also be able to get more done. Getting more done will simultaneously mean you have less to worry about. You will create a positive cycle that compounds the more you can induce your own state of relaxation.

A Tool for Relaxation

Simply sit, stand, lay down or whatever is most realistic and relaxing at the moment. Breathe in deeply. Exhale all of the air out. Repeat and simply feel. Inhale and exhale. As you exhale, imagine all of the tension leaving your body and mind. It is simply melting away. Imagine yourself standing on a bridge over a bubbling brook or a steady river. Imagine that all of your worries are simply slipping away into the cold water below. The water neutralizes them and they just wash away, leaving only a state of calm. Breathe deeply until you feel better.

You can practice deep breathing anywhere. At your desk, at home, in bed or even while driving. (Be sure to stay alert and with your eyes open though if you are driving. Simply allow yourself to breathe in and out deeply while concentrating on the road.)

Other Great Ways to Reduce Stress

Other ways to reduce stress are exercise, spending time with friends, watching funny movies or short videos on YouTube, doing something you enjoy, reading a good book, playing with your kids or your pets. Basically anything that you like doing will help you to relieve stress.

Once you are adept at getting yourself to relax in even the most demanding situations (remember to breathe deeply before going into an important meeting or job interview), you will find it easier to lose weight and all of the other techniques you put to work for you will become more effective.

Healthy Habit #1:

Instead of worrying, breathe deeply! You can never get to much oxygen. Practice the simple art of deep breathing.

Chapter 2: Get moving: the best exercises

Everyone knows that moving the body burns calories and assists in weight loss. But there is more to it than that.

Movement, especially jumping, gets the lymph moving. The lymph is a system right below the skin that processes waste. Unlike the blood, it does not circulate automatically. We need to move the body to get the lymph to move and to process and to get wastes out. Anything that involves jumping is great toward this end.

When you wake up in the morning, try hopping up and down 20-30 times. Then do 30 jumping jacks. This will get your heart rate going, your blood pumping, and will activate your lymph system. A well-functioning lymph system helps to keep you from getting sick as often since it can process wastes and enable the immune system to effectively neutralize invaders. Many people have a slow lymph system and find it difficult to lose weight. Hop up and down every day to help along the lymph. You will work your heart, increase oxygen to your lungs and cells, and help the lymph out.

Do What You Love

From there, we can say that the best exercises are those you enjoy! Find something you are really passionate about and then do that A LOT. You don't want to feel like your work out is a drag. Often, the problem with fitness studio exercising is that you get bored staring at the treadmill. If you really like this style of working out, that's great. Try listening to your favorite music while you work out so that you get energized by it. An upbeat song can make the difference between simply dragging yourself through the exercises and doing them with power and enthusiasm.

This takes us back to the stress aspect from Chapter 1: doing what you like to do reduces stress. Forcing yourself to do something you don't like will just make you feel worse. So be sure to find some sport, physical activity or workout that you love to do. Challenge yourself so that you can grow and improve, but don't overwhelm yourself. If you're into running and jogging, slowly increase the intensity of your run each day. Don't exhaust yourself, and don't bore yourself. Find the balance and keep that balance.

Some exercises that are timeless in their effectiveness include crunches, pushups, jumping jacks, sit-ups, pull-ups, weight lifting and running.

The current favorite among personal trainers and fitness experts is the burpee.

Burpees

What is the burpee? This explosive exercise works the whole body, gets the heart rate going and is extremely effective in toning muscles and improving cardio condition. How is it done? It combines the push-up and jumping quickly to form an excellent exercise.

First, do a push-up. Bring yourself close to the ground, then raise yourself up, keeping the body straight. Now jump up to your feet and jump into the air as far off the ground as you can raising your arms over the head. (You can clap your hands when you jump up if you like). Repeat this quickly and explosively as many times as you can. Combine the burpee with the simple plank to really target your abs.

The plank

The plank is a familiar exercise from Yoga and other fitness programs.

Simply hold your body in the raised push-up stance. Keep the body straight and breathe deeply. Feel the burn in your abs. Stay here for a minute. Then switch back to burpees for two minutes. Repeat this exercise series three times or more if you need a challenge.

What else is there?

There is so much out there that you can choose from to get your body moving. You don't need to join a gym to get a good workout, but this is a good solution for a lot of people. Using equipment allows you to track the miles you've run, the amount of weights you can lift, and there are people you can ask for help when operating the equipment. A gym workout is the most fun in the presence of a friend, or with your favorite music playing on an ipod or other mp3 player.

Other sports you can do include running in the woods. The woods is an excellent place to run since the uneven paths force you to use parts of your leg muscles you otherwise might not be able to target as effectively. Tree roots and bushes also force you to be alert and watch where you are going. This trains alertness which is good for the mind and for the senses. There is a lot of fresh air in the woods from the trees, and quality air is essential for health.

Try swimming, try team sports, go dancing, try belly dancing or other types of dancing. Whatever gets you feeling good and inspired and moving , that's what you need to stick with.

Another positive point of exercise is that it causes the brain to release endorphins. Endorphins are feel-good hormones. This also indirectly affects your ability to effectively lose weight. If you feel good, you aren't stressing. A lack of stress means a lack of cortisol. A lack of cortisol means easier weight loss.

Healthy Habit #2 :
Instead of sitting down on the couch after work when you feel stressed or tired, get moving! This will increase your energy, decrease stress and help you to lose weight! Whenever you feel stressed, sad or angry, go running or do some sport or physical activity that you love to more healthily deal with the demands of life.

Chapter 3: Drinks for Fitness

Many people consume an unbelievable amount of calories just with drinks. They can't get full this way, and they fill themselves with sugar that is then stored as fat.

Quit the fruit juice and soda. You may understand that soda needs to go, but the juice may come as a surprise. Fruit contains sugar. Though a healthier form of sugar than that found in soda, it still gets stored as fat in the body. To get the vitamins and health benefits of fruit, replace the juice drink with an orange or an apple (organic is best). The full fruit provides you with fiber that will help you to feel full and prevent you from overeating. The sugar in fruit juice stimulates the appetite and can lead to overeating.

Instead of Juice and Soda

If you love the fizzy taste from the carbonation in soda, try replacing the soda with Kombucha. Kombucha is made from cultured tea and provides the body with probiotics. It tastes great, is a fizzy drink and is much healthier than soda (it is also free of sugar!)

Finally, to quench your thirst and flush toxins out of the body you need to drink PLENTY of good water. Make sure it is chlorine and fluoride free, use a filter or reverse osmosis to get the best possible water. If you don't have access to this, boil your water or buy water in glass bottles. Make sure you drink at least 2 liters a day. A great way to start your day is by drinking a glass of lemon water. Simply squeeze some lemon into a cup of warm water and drink right away. Drink two if so desired. This helps balance the pH of the body and nourishes the system with vitamin C and refreshing water.

Healthy Habit #3:
Eat fruit instead of drinking fruit juice. Drink Kombucha instead of soda. To quench thirst, drink water.

Chapter 4: Yummy! What to Eat

There are so many diets out there promising to be the best there is. To keep it simple we can say, reduce portions to lose weight and reduce calories. It can be as easy as that!

But to go deeper in and eat for health and wellness in addition to weighing less you will want to reduce your intake of sugar. Avoid all processed sugar and processed foods. Real, whole foods are what you want to stick with. Fruits, vegetables, whole grains (in moderation), coconut oil, organic butter, olive oil, nuts, lean meat like chicken, turkey and fish are all delicious and healthy. Make your diet mostly consist of vegetables. Serve them with good fats like coconut oil or organic butter.

This is important because some vitamins are only fat soluble. For your body to be able to absorb these vitamins, you need to eat them with some form of fat. Coconut oil, butter and cold-pressed olive oil are always a good choice. You can also eat a salad with olive oil and apple cider vinegar. Apple cider vinegar tastes great and helps to stimulate weight loss. A small portion of meat or fish provides you with the protein you need. A handful of nuts in between meals is an excellent way to stave off hunger and keeps the

17

metabolism going while supplying the system with a slew of vitamins and minerals. Fruit is sugar, so be sure to consume only moderately.

Veggies and More Veggies

It is often thought that you can never eat too many fruits and veggies. We absolutely encourage you to eat vegetables with every meal, get your greens and enjoy. However, you want to limit your fruit consumption. Sugar is sugar, no matter the source and it is a culprit when it comes to weight gain. Eat an apple or a handful of berries with your breakfast accompanying organic yoghurt, but don't snack on fruit in between meals. You will make yourself hungrier and your body will turn the sugar into fat, especially if you have a desk job. A couple grapes before exercising is OK, but you want to eat as little sugar as you can.

Cheese, Please?

Goat and sheep cheese are better for the stomach. Eat a bit of chevre cheese with a salad along with sunflower seeds to get protein and help yourself feel full. It is high in fat but is easier for the body to break down and doesn't cause cravings the same way that cow's milk cheese often does. (The higher amount of milk sugar in an aged cow's cheese such as cheddar leads to cravings that can throw a diet off). Feta

18

cheese is delicious as part of a Greek salad with black olives, cucumbers and tomatoes and olive oil.

Healthy Habit # 4 :
Reduce portions to reduce weight. Eat only whole foods. Don't eat processed food, and limit your sugar intake.

Chapter 5: Recipes for that Flat Stomach

In the last chapter, we talked a lot about what you can and can't eat. Now we are going to provide you with some good recipes so you can cook your own delicious and healthy meals.

Breakfast:
Green Smoothie

Ingredients:

Half an avocado

A handful of strawberries or raspberries

A handful of baby spinach

One quarter of a banana

A few chunks of frozen mango

2 cups of sugar free, carageenen free almond milk

In a blender, combine all of the ingredients. Blend until smooth. Drink right away. (Tip: chew your smoothie to activate the digestive juices so that you can properly digest the smoothie. Chewing activates the digestive system.)

The great thing with green smoothies is you can switch around ingredients, add supplement powder (Amazing Grass makes delicious Superfood powders you can add to smoothies for a chocolate, orange or berry taste. They are organic and sugar free). Try switching out mango for cherries, or switch out spinach with Swiss chard. Avocado gives the smoothie a creamy consistency, but you can't taste it in your smoothie.

Lunch:

Take Me to Work Salad

Ingredients:

A head of green lettuce

Half a cucumber

One tomato

Half an avocado

Two tablespoons of olive oil

Salt and pepper to taste

A bit of feta cheese

Wash all the vegetables well. Cut up the lettuce into bite sized bits. Slice the cucumber, slice the tomato or dice it. Slice the avocado. Place all of the vegetables in a transportable container (Tupperware, etc). Then top with the olive oil, salt and pepper and cheese. Make it in the morning before you go to work or the night before. (It's super quick and easy)

Carrot Ginger Soup

4 organic carrots

A bit of ginger root

Salt and pepper

Fresh herbs (oregano, basil, thyme or whatever is available)

A pinch of garlic and onion powder

Peel and cut the carrots up into bits. Boil a pot of water and add the carrots. Cook until the vegetables are tender. Then drain some of the water so just enough remains to cover the carrots (but not too much or your soup will be too watery). Reduce the water to low heat. Peel and dice the ginger. Add the ginger to the carrots. Then add the fresh herbs as well as the garlic and onion powder. Turn off the heat and mash the carrots with a hand-masher (a fork will do in a pinch) or a hand held mixer. You can add a bit of coconut oil and coconut cream if you would like a richer flavor. Salt and pepper to taste.

Dinner:

Rice, veggies and fish

Ingredients:

1 cup of brown rice

2 cups of broccoli, carrots and red bell peppers

A small cut of salmon or cod

A dash of soy sauce to season

A bit of pepper to taste

Boil the brown rice according to package directions. Steam the broccoli, carrots and peppers. Bake the salmon or cod with a bit of olive oil. Serve the fish with a squeeze of lemon if so desired. Combine the rice and vegetables in a dish when they are finished. Add the dash of soy sauce and pepper. Finally, top with the fish and enjoy! Double the ingredients to cook for more than one person.

Grilled Veggies and Chicken

Ingredients:

Your choice of vegetables (zucchini, bell pepper, eggplant, mushrooms, onions are all great on the grill)

Organic chicken

Marinate the vegetables and chicken in olive oil and then grill them to perfection. Serve them with some pesto and feta cheese for a delicious dinner that's perfect eaten outdoors in the summertime.

Habit # 5:
Instead of cooking the same old thing, search the Internet for healthy recipes. Healthy salads, lean meat, lots of steamed veggies should comprise your delicious and easy meals. Salads are fast to prepare and are nourishing and healthy and conducive to weight loss. Avocado, goat cheese, fish and lean meat are filling and great in small portions. Cooking your own food will give you greater control over what you put into your body. As a result, you will have greater control over your own health and your life!

Chapter 6: Supplements: Yes or No? (Yes! The right ones)

You've probably read or heard that diet pills are unsafe and unhealthy. That's true. They also are a type of cheating, wouldn't you say? Isn't it better to turn your life around for the long term? The good habits you create now will help you build a long and good life. Diet pills on the other hand corrode the health, create dependence and cause weight gain once you go off of them. Then it's difficult to lose the weight gained after going off of the diet pills.

Does this mean there is nothing you can do to make losing weight easier? Of course not! There's a lot you can do that's healthy and beneficial for you overall.

Green Tea: Energy and Health!!
One powerful herb to include on your weight loss journey is green tea. The natural caffeine helps to suppress the appetite while giving energy. In addition, the antioxidants in green tea neutralize free radicals, thus keeping you healthier overall and keeping you from getting sick as often.

Green tea is also said to help whiten the teeth and is good for the gums. A cup of green tea in the morning with breakfast gives you energy and is healthier and better than coffee (especially for the teeth). You can drink green tea throughout the day, but you will want to ease up before the afternoon so that you can sleep in the evening! Tea has less caffeine than coffee, but it will still keep you up at night if you drink too much of it.

Lemon Water: Oh Yes!
Lemon water helps to detoxify the body, and as such is also a powerful tool toward losing weight. It flushes out toxins and regulates the pH.

Plain old ordinary water is also helpful in losing weight. If you drink lots of water, you will feel less hungry and be less likely to overindulge in any type of food. Try to drink more than 2 liters of water every day, in the best quality of water you can find.

Aloe vera juice is good for the digestive system. It helps to clean out the digestive tract, keeps fungus at bay and flushes out impurities. Be sure to drink plenty of water with aloe vera. You will notice you have to go to the bathroom more often, but this is a sign it's working! You want the bad stuff out, not in.

Other Herbs
Another herb that is great for the digestive system and for awakening energy is ginger. It increases the circulation with its spicy goodness. You can add it to

soups (such as carrot soup with coconut milk) or even to smoothies. It eases the stomach, helps against nausea and gives energy. Feeling energized helps to keep you from overeating. Improved circulation means better health.

Other supplements that are good for health in general are vitamins and minerals. You will want to make sure they are sourced from organic food and are not synthetic. Synthetic vitamins do more harm than good. Food-based vitamin tablets are natural and easy for the body to work with.

Tip 6: Green tea (as a drink or in tablet form) is an excellent and natural supplement to help you effectively lose weight!

Chapter 7: Maintain with a Healthy Body and Mind

Once you have reached your ideal weight, you will need to maintain your ideal weight. How is this accomplished? Things like chocolates and French fries are so tempting and they are everywhere, consumed by many. How can you keep from gaining weight in the midst of inner pressure?

The main approach is to recognize your diet and exercise program as not a temporary change, but as a real and significant lifestyle change that you are committed to for the rest of your life. Sacrificing the enjoyment of unhealthy foods for your health, well-being, happiness and self-confidence is a small price to pay for such a huge gain. Remember, no food tastes as good as you feel fitting into all of your clothes and looking great when you look in the mirror. You also reduce your chances of heart disease, cancer and other illnesses by reducing your weight. So this is something that deserves an overall change of mind along with the change of body.

That said, it may feel too extreme for some to completely say goodbye to cheesecake and chocolates. In some rare circumstances, you may allow yourself to enjoy a small piece of cake, a bit of ice cream, or one piece of expensive luxury chocolate. If you only allow yourself to eat the best and most expensive sweets, your finances will also demand that you don't overdo it!

An obstacle some people report when trying to lose weight and gain health is that of a lack of money, living on a strict budget and being unable to afford healthy foods. Healthy food does NOT need to be expensive. Yes, it is easy to spend a lot of money at a shop like Whole Foods Market, but it is also possible to buy inexpensive but great and nourishing ingredients to making delicious dinners that will enable you to lose weight while providing you with the vitamins and minerals you need.

For example, carrots are very inexpensive and are full of nutrition. An avocado is usually very expensive, but if you buy them while they are on sale and then eat half for lunch and half for dinner you can save a lot of money. You can also determine your meal plans by seeing what is on sale that week and then plan your meals according to that.

A good place to find less expensive produce is the local farmer's market. Since you are buying things direct, you cut out the middle man and thus eliminate costs. You can also inquire as to growing methods and ask for advice in preparing the food you buy. You are also doing something good for your community by supporting a small business (the farm). Thus, you can feel good about yourself on various levels.

Try prioritizing health over other things. If you give up buying sweets, you will have more money for healthy veggies. If you quit drinking, you can spend that money on healthier foods. You can find some area of your life where you are maybe not spending as wisely as you could be, cut that habit out and replace that with the habit of buying healthy fruits and vegetables.

Exercising doesn't have to cost anything at all. Sure, you can spend loads of cash on fancy equipment, expensive trips to compete in marathons, scuba diving lessons and so on, but you don't need to! A jog around the block is free. A hike in the woods costs nothing (except maybe the gas to get there if you don't live next to the woods). Swimming in lakes and the sea is free. Dancing to videos on the Internet is free.

Turning on your favorite music and doing interval training costs nothing. Jumping jacks in the morning cost nothing. There's so much you can do that costs next to nothing, or is totally free. Concentrate on doing good for yourself, and the rest will fall into place no matter how small your budget is!

The mind is the most important factor in all of this. If you really want to be healthy and fit, you will make it happen. Books such as this one guide you on your path, but they are useless if you haven't made up your mind to really lose the weight, really get in shape and follow through with it. You need to have the motivation that comes from within to turn your life around. The power is yours, no matter how hard things seem. It really just comes to simply switching bad habits out with good ones.

Replace Bad Habits with Good Habits
Here are some more bad habits you can replace with great ones.

Sitting on the couch too long: Replace this habit with a walk around the block. Look at the sunset, pick out constellations in the sky or take your. If you want a more challenging workout, run around the block. Stretch your muscles, get breathing, have fun and see more of the world!

Getting cravings to eat unhealthy snacks: Drink two glasses of water and see if that helps. If it doesn't help go for a walk or do some pushups and then drink another glass of water. Chances are, the cravings will be gone. If you are truly hungry, eat a handful of almonds or make a healthy meal (if it's mealtime).

Snacking too much: Instead of eating big snacks like bread, chips, rolls, pastries, etc reduce your snacks to just a handful of nuts (almonds, cashews, walnuts, etc).

Overeating at mealtimes: If you are single and live alone, cook just enough for that one meal. If you want to cook for the next day (for something to take to work) then be sure to put away the portion you are saving. Pack it up and put it in the refrigerator BEFORE you sit down to eat the meal at hand. If you live in the context of a family, serve everyone else first, then take your share. Be sure to not put too much on your plate. NEVER eat seconds! Completely cut that habit out of your life.

Craving desert: Instead of eating a full-on desert, try drinking a cup of tea sweetened with stevia and with a splash of sugar free almond milk. This will give your "sweet tooth" what it wants without packing on the calories.

Feeling overwhelmed by the thought of exercise: Start out slow and increase just a bit each day. For example, on day one do just 10 jumping jacks. The next day, do 12. Then increase by two each day. Do just enough to get yourself moving in the beginning. Soon you will find you feel better after exercising and will want to do it more often. You will get the urge to push yourself. This will come with time, so there's no need to rush. It is NOT healthy to try to go from being a couch potato to a marathon runner. Take it slow, but consistently do more and more each day that passes.

Putting loads of sugar and milk in your coffee: If you must drink coffee, stop drinking sugar and milk with it. Instead, use sugar free almond milk in your coffee and sweeten it with stevia. Stevia is a calorie free plant that tastes naturally sweet. It is completely healthy, tasty and excellent for those trying to lose weight. Replace cow's milk with almond milk and sugar with stevia.

Eating too much at parties: Instead of joining the pig-out fest at parties and celebrations, eat a little bit before you leave. Then when you get to the party, sample just a little bit instead of eating large portions. Get just enough so you have the taste, but don't eat to the point where you want more and more and find it difficult to stop.

Craving bread in the morning: The morning is a time where many people eat too many starches and carbohydrates. Instead of blasting the body with what it doesn't need, give it the nutrition it needs in the form of a tasty and filling green smoothie. The vegetables and the fruit have lots of fiber which will fill you up. The natural sugars in the fruit will give you an energy boost without making you feel crazy for more, and the vegetables will give you nutrition. Another good breakfast is organic yoghurt. This has protein and probiotics which help make you feel full and assist gut health. Instead of bread, go for a smoothie or yoghurt.

Lacking the energy and the willpower: Everyone goes through times where they have less energy and less willpower than otherwise. This is totally normal. Don't let yourself succumb to the lazy feeling though, and gently push yourself to work out. Be gentle with yourself, accept that you don't feel great that day, but stick to your healthy routine. Once you have made healthy eating and exercise a habit and a routine, it won't be hard at all to work through the tired feeling.

If you suspect you are getting ill and really don't feel well, consider seeing a doctor or take it easy that day. You don't want to injure yourself.

Conclusion

For every bad habit, there's a great habit you can replace it with. Turning things around for the better is about doing good for yourself and making health and wellness a routine and a positive habit in your life. Drinking lots of water, eating only nourishing foods, working out regularly and keeping a good attitude are the foundation for a long and happy life. Once you start out on this path, you will never want to stop! Exercise boosts the body with endorphins and healthy food gives the cells what they need. This is what you need in your life. Best of luck! You can do it!!

www.ingramcontent.com/pod-product-compliance
Lightning Source LLC
Chambersburg PA
CBHW070936290526
45795CB00003B/1037